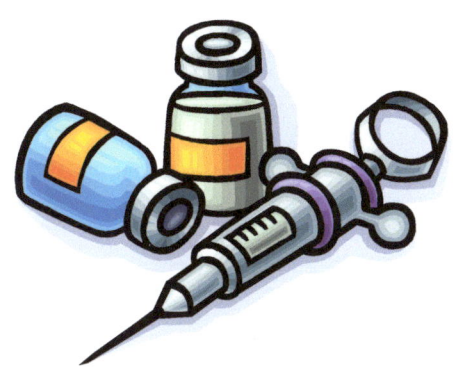

Blood Sugar and Insulin Log

This Notebook Belongs to:

_____

Month _____ to Month _____ Year _____

For my mom, Iva

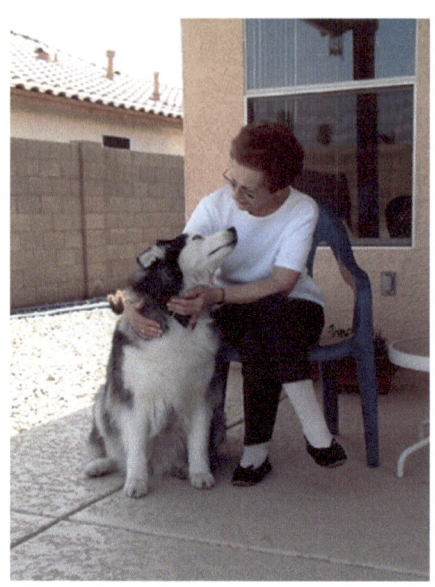

Written and Published by
Claudia Barros MSN RN CCM
7821 North 173rd Avenue
Waddell AZ 85355

Do not duplicate, disseminate, or appropriate this
book without written permission of the author.

Insulin Basics

Your doctor has started you on a Subcutaneous Insulin Sliding Scale. This insulin is short-acting.

The scale may be Mild, Moderate or Aggressive depending on your blood sugar readings and your insulin needs. Over time, your doctor may adjust your sliding scale.

You may also be placed on a basal dose of long-acting insulin to help regulate your blood sugar. This dose will be determined by your doctor and may be adjusted as your blood sugar control improves.

Your goal is to assist your doctor in maintaining an accurate record of your blood sugar and insulin doses administered. The key is to try to keep your blood sugar below 200 mg/dl and above 80 mg/dl.

Track all of your blood sugar readings and how much insulin is administered. Make a note of the time of day and whether you ate a meal.

The Blood Sugar and Insulin Log is a convenient tool for efficiently tracking all of this important information.

Checking your Blood Sugar

- ♥ Use your blood sugar test strips and lancets for testing your blood sugar
- ♥ Check your blood sugar before every meal and at bedtime
- ♥ For example: 7 am, 12 noon, 4 pm, and 10 pm
- ♥ Draw-up your short-acting insulin per the sliding scale
- ♥ Inject into skin before each meal
- ♥ Eat within 15 minutes of administering insulin
- ♥ Track your information in the log
- ♥ Consume a Diabetic Diet for breakfast, lunch and dinner
- ♥ If your doctor has you on a long-acting insulin administer this medication after checking your blood sugar at night
- ♥ Eat a snack before bedtime
- ♥ Have your doctor check your Hemoglobin A1C every 3 months

Sliding Scale Samples

These insulin sliding scales are samples ONLY. Please follow the Sliding Scale ordered by your doctor.

MILD Short-Actin Insulin Sliding Scale

150-199	2 units
200-249	4 units
250-299	6 units
300-349	8 units
Greater than 349	10 units

MODERATE Short-Actin Insulin Sliding Scale

150-199	4 units
200-249	8 units
250-299	10 units
300-349	12 units
Greater than 349	16 units

AGGRESSIVE Short-Actin Insulin Sliding Scale

150-199	8 units
200-249	12 units
250-299	16 units
300-349	20 units
Greater than 349	24 units

IN ALL CASES
If your blood sugar is less than 60 or greater than 400 --- Call your doctor immediately

Your Sliding Scale

Please enter the Short-Acting Sliding Scale ordered by your doctor HERE.

Circle one:
MILD   MODERATE   AGGRESSIVE

Blood Sugar Range	Units to Administer

Insulin Type	Dose & Frequency

Managing Low Blood Sugar

Signs and Symptoms of Low Blood Sugar

- ♥ Nervous
- ♥ Trembling
- ♥ Dizzy
- ♥ Weak
- ♥ Headache
- ♥ Hungry
- ♥ Nausea
- ♥ Pale
- ♥ Sweaty
- ♥ Blurred vision
- ♥ Irritable
- ♥ Confused
- ♥ Tingling mouth or tongue
- ♥ Slowed responses

How to Treat

Treat blood sugar less than 70 mg/dl with or without symptoms.

Treat blood sugar less than 80 mg/dl with symptoms.

Treat by taking a fast-acting carbohydrate

- ♥ 3 glucose tablets
- ♥ 4 ounces fruit juice
- ♥ 8 ounces skim milk
- ♥ 6 ounces regular soda
- ♥ 3 graham crackers
- ♥ 6 saltine crackers

Recheck your blood sugar in 15 minutes

Once your blood sugar is over 80 mg/dl eat a snack or meal.

Call your doctor and let him know that you needed to treat a low blood sugar ...

If you become unconscious, someone needs to call 911.

When to Call

Call your doctor immediately when you
- ♥ Become symptomatic
- ♥ Have to treat your low blood sugar
- ♥ Are unable to eat
- ♥ Develop persistent nausea, vomiting or diarrhea
- ♥ Develop a fever greater than 101 degrees Fahrenheit (38.3 degrees Celsius)
- ♥ Have a change in level of consciousness
- ♥ If your blood sugar is less than 60 or greater than 400
- ♥ Have blood sugar readings less than 70 mg/dl or greater than 300 mg/dl on 3 consecutive measurements

Giving Insulin

Equipment
Blood sugar monitor, strips and lancets. Make sure you have purchased the correct syringes and insulin vials or pen.

- ♥ Examine your vials or pens for contamination
- ♥ Store and handle your insulin as instructed
- ♥ Rapid or short-acting insulin does not need to be mixed
- ♥ For intermediate or long-acting insulin, roll the insulin bottle between your hands to mix

Review and practice insulin injection technique. Insulin is normally injected under the skin with a very small needle. Insulin can also be taken with an insulin pen. Practice …

- ♥ Nurse on patient
- ♥ Patient on self
- ♥ Significant other on patient

Administration Sites

- ♥ The upper arm --- works at medium speed
- ♥ The front and side of the thighs --- work slowest
- ♥ The abdomen --- works fastest
- ♥ Rotate your sites every day

Technique
- ♥ Wash your hands before and after administering insulin
- ♥ Clean your skin with alcohol
- ♥ Grab a fold of skin and inject the insulin at a 90-degree angle
- ♥ If you are thin, you may need to pinch the skin and inject the insulin at a 45-degree angle

Disposal of Needles
- ♥ Think safety
- ♥ Place each used syringe in a proper needle holder for disposal
- ♥ Do not throw used syringes in the regular trash
- ♥ Used syringes are medical waste and should be disposed of in a medical waste container

ADMINISTRATION CHECK LIST

- ☐ Wash your hands
- ☐ Do you have the right Insulin?
- ☐ Check the expiration date
- ☐ Check insulin closely for clumps or crystals
- ☐ Does the bottle need to be mixed?
- ☐ Get the right syringe and needle or use an Insulin Pen as prescribed by your doctor
- ☐ Inject air into the bottle (if you are using a syringe and needle)
- ☐ Draw-up or Dial-up the correct dose
- ☐ Remove air bubbles (if you are using a syringe and needle)
- ☐ Choose appropriate site
- ☐ Pinch an inch of skin
- ☐ Choose correct angle of injection (90 degrees or 45 degrees)
- ☐ Press injection site gently after withdrawing needle
- ☐ Check site for signs of infection (warmth, redness, or yellow drainage)
- ☐ Document the date, time, blood sugar reading and the time you ate
- ☐ Document the type of insulin (rapid, short-acting, intermediate, or long-acting) and the dose you administered

DAILY LOG

Date	Time	Blood Sugar	Insulin Type and Dose	Meal Time

Date	Time	Blood Sugar	Insulin Type and Dose	Meal Time

Date	Time	Blood Sugar	Insulin Type and Dose	Meal Time

Date	Time	Blood Sugar	Insulin Type and Dose	Meal Time

Date	Time	Blood Sugar	Insulin Type and Dose	Meal Time

Date	Time	Blood Sugar	Insulin Type and Dose	Meal Time

Date	Time	Blood Sugar	Insulin Type and Dose	Meal Time

Date	Time	Blood Sugar	Insulin Type and Dose	Meal Time

Date	Time	Blood Sugar	Insulin Type and Dose	Meal Time

Date	Time	Blood Sugar	Insulin Type and Dose	Meal Time

Date	Time	Blood Sugar	Insulin Type and Dose	Meal Time

Date	Time	Blood Sugar	Insulin Type and Dose	Meal Time

Date	Time	Blood Sugar	Insulin Type and Dose	Meal Time

Date	Time	Blood Sugar	Insulin Type and Dose	Meal Time

Date	Time	Blood Sugar	Insulin Type and Dose	Meal Time

Date	Time	Blood Sugar	Insulin Type and Dose	Meal Time

Date	Time	Blood Sugar	Insulin Type and Dose	Meal Time

Date	Time	Blood Sugar	Insulin Type and Dose	Meal Time

Date	Time	Blood Sugar	Insulin Type and Dose	Meal Time

Date	Time	Blood Sugar	Insulin Type and Dose	Meal Time

Date	Time	Blood Sugar	Insulin Type and Dose	Meal Time

Date	Time	Blood Sugar	Insulin Type and Dose	Meal Time

Date	Time	Blood Sugar	Insulin Type and Dose	Meal Time

Date	Time	Blood Sugar	Insulin Type and Dose	Meal Time

Date	Time	Blood Sugar	Insulin Type and Dose	Meal Time

Date	Time	Blood Sugar	Insulin Type and Dose	Meal Time

Date	Time	Blood Sugar	Insulin Type and Dose	Meal Time

Date	Time	Blood Sugar	Insulin Type and Dose	Meal Time

Notes:

www.ingramcontent.com/pod-product-compliance
Lightning Source LLC
Chambersburg PA
CBHW041114180526
45172CB00001B/253